A TO Z
MINIMALISM

LIVE SIMPLE
CLEAR YOUR MIND

LISA BOND

Table of Contents

Copyright © 2017 by sbBooks

Lisa Bond
    lisa@atozlisabond.com

    www.atozlisabond.com

Introduction

We've all heard it time and time again. Keep it simple, stupid! What does that even mean, right?! Well, when we're talking about things like living a Minimalist lifestyle, it *is* that simple. We're not talking about just ridding your home of a bunch of clutter or quelling that innate need to watch every *Real Housewives* episode as it is released, but what we mean is taking it to the basement level of your life in general. Remodel everything right down to how you behave and view the world.

Don't allow yourself to continue as a slave to technology, trends, antiquated attitudes that are like dogma chaining you to complicated ideas and causing unhappiness for falling short of impossibly high expectations that people can sometimes place on themselves. This is not only a constant let down, but it buys into a capitalist ideal that is voraciously insatiable. Above all else, the idea of Minimalism allows you to remain unencumbered by the mentality that everything in life must be so complex or hard to take on. And why should it be? Isn't life hard enough with all the things our careers, relationships and mundane circumstances throw at us?

Yes, Minimalism will mean dumping off possessions, but it's also dumping some of the mental garbage cluttering our minds –a breaking free of the world that says you must have 4 social media accounts and 20 passwords on digital media. The inner voice providing piece in a world of wo-car homes, where keeping up with the Joneses bleeds into our spirituality, how we raise our children and every other facet of our cultural being.

The truth is we do not need all the things. We don't need all these attitudes. We can break free; it's freeing and lightening to the load we all must bear. So if life is already so difficult and tedious, why not give it a shot? There is nothing but things to gain from trying out a new perspective.

Join in and see how unhindered you can become with a few minor tweaks to your way of thinking. It's definitely not just about possessions, and a Minimalist lifestyle and way of thinking could be just what you needed all along.

Chapter One: Minimalism Beyond Throwing out Your HD TV

That's correct! Minimalism is so much more than having a massive Craigslist-fest to rid your home and life of your TV set, vehicles and endless parade of possessions. It can be a great start for those who passionately delve into a new mindset without the need to hang onto *stuff*. However, we need to back up for a second and examine Minimalism further for you to really understand what this lifestyle concept actually means.

It's going to mean a lot of introspection -soul-searching, if you will. This is not just a home décor scheme or choosing to bike to work. You should be committed to a change in your thought patterns and the way you approach life in general. Hold onto your hat –even if you think you need to ditch that too because this is going to be a game-changer!

Defining the Minimalist Concept

Again, reducing your load of possessions isn't a bad place to start when adopting the Minimalist concept into your life. However, this isn't where the concept begins and ends. This is, by far, the largest misconception, which makes people often miss the entire point or ditch the lifestyle altogether after all too short a period of time to really come to grips with what it means to become a true Minimalist. So what is Minimalism?

Simply put, Minimalists seek to declutter their lives by lightening the load on their minds and souls. It's about simplifying your life from the inside out. Leaving behind the things in your mind that make life complicated –resisting the urge to fill life with things but rather fill them with experiences that can be of use to oneself in the grips of a society that has too much to think about, commit their individual lives to and more.

Start off by thinking about the things that cause you stress in your life. Is your job a major stumbling block when it comes to dedicating your life and energy to what you personally believe really matters most? Do you have too much debt? Are you spending too much time with people that aren't as worthwhile as those who matter most fall by the wayside? Do you find your spirituality suffering as you put the daily grind (whatever that means to you) in front of your mental and emotional wellbeing? This is all important stuff that's waving a red flag in your face as you attempt to plod through another day.

Perhaps buying into the Capitalist lifestyle isn't even the issue. Maybe the things you choose to spend your hard-earned wage on should simply be of more personal value and less monetary. In fact, even expensive things can be okay to enjoy as long as they bring you joy.

Okay, I have to admit, seems fairly loosely defined, doesn't it? You bet! I guess that's the whole point though. Don't be locked in by one ideal or another that defines you or creates a prison within itself. That's completely contrary to the whole idea. Yes, be friendly to the earth, create less waste, be frugal, go for quality over quantity in your personal relationships and definitely don't live a cluttered life, but above all else, do not feel locked into one definition or another. That would be problematic on its own.

Even with this very idea being intrinsic to the inner workings of Minimalism, you are going to want to keep a few points in mind when exploring the concept.

1. Keep uncluttered surroundings.
2. Keep an uncluttered mind through practices like yoga or meditation.
3. Eliminate stressors in your environment such as toxic people or negative attitudes.
4. Explore paths of spirituality that take joy in small and simple tenets.
5. Take joy in nature.
6. Live greener.
7. Do not let the things you own own you.
8. Try to work in a career that provides you with more spare time or personal fulfilment.
9. Stop trying to be all things to all people.
10. Allow yourself more time to do what you enjoy.

If you can keep to these important and very simple concepts, you've got a fairly good handle on a Minimalist lifestyle, which can absolutely provide you with all the happiness you need. Let's face it, there isn't any amount of money, possessions or friends that can provide that for you. It's going to come from within and from yourself or not at all.

Sometimes You Must Put on The Blinders

One of the more challenging parts of Minimalism has to be blocking out the negativity. You bet! We all have a world of it swirling inside our heads from time to time. Self-doubt, depression and lack of focus are just some of the major challenges that plague us most; there's also a huge world of negative thought patterns and other ghosts *out there* to help deter us as well. Every time that we watch TV, for instance, there's a TV series on about crime, a talk show about the human condition and how we've failed one another and a million news stories waiting to let us know how horrible we are to each other.

We get in our cars or on our bikes and get honked at or flipped off, sit down at our desks in an office full of people who want to complain about their kids, spouse or boss, and then we have to work with people who also seem to regularly have a bone to pick with our companies or the world at large. To be honest, there are some days that are hard to see anything good about the world –nevermind anything simplistic.

That's a great place to start though! Start with putting on your mental ear muffs when you go on your break and someone wants to bitch and complain about the customer they just spoke with. You're on your break, for Pete's sake! The complaint department is closed. If the news is depressing, then why are you watching it? Shut it off after you've seen the weather and sports. Mute it if the top stories always revolve around people hurting each other. Watch shows that lift people up or make you laugh instead of dark and sinister tales of backstabbing and the macabre.

Hey, sometimes in life, you just gotta put on the blinders and forget that garbage exists to keep an upbeat outlook. No one else is going to block that stuff out for you; especially in such a small world with technology reporting across the globe on every little tragedy and wrong the world has to offer and report on or where profit and interest seem to be focused mostly on the shocking or horrible in the world. You wouldn't think it would be that easy –for some people, it isn't. But it can be if you are really committed to feeling less weighed down by all that emotional heaviness. Because that's exactly what it is: heaviness you elect to place on your proverbial shoulders.

You'll more likely find that with all that nasty stuff eradicated from your surroundings, you have more time to spend focusing on yourself and your happiness instead, which is fantastic! Who wouldn't want that? I don't think I've ever heard anyone say: "That guy's such a downer, I love hanging out with him!". Why do you think that is? It takes a lot of energy out of people to hang around the Debbie Downer in a group, which goes same for shows, places and situations of the same gravity.

So start by blocking this stuff out or at least keep these types of moods to a minimum, and you'll be well on your way!

Chapter Two: Spiritual Practices that Encourage Minimalism

If anything is an excellent teacher of how to live a Minimalist lifestyle, there is nothing better than spirituality. There are many different types of spirituality out in the world that aptly demonstrate what it means to eradicate daily external distraction and all sorts of clutter from one's life. Even the far-reaching corners of the earth's aborigine sects of tribal spirituality show how this can be achieved.

There are more popular and well-known religions and spiritual practices that also show how this works, which can easily be examined both here and in your own studies. Heck, even looking through a few articles on each of them and their specific facets is effective in showing what can be done to eliminate all the 'noise' in your life. Here, you will see the most well-known of these and some of the best ways they use Minimalist trains of thought to achieve particular goals.

Monastic Vows of Silence

Okay, so despite popular belief, it isn't one religion or another or its vows that say you have to devote yourself to silence. However, there are many of them and their devotional exercises that exact themselves through things like the infamous *Vow of Silence*. This happens in Christianity, Judaism, Hinduism and Buddhism but other religions too where a devout member of the order will maintain silence at certain times of day or in certain areas of the monastery to observe their work well. This can also be a huge part of what they need to do in order to attain the goal for whichever activity they are searching to fulfill as is the case with activities like meditation.

This is absolutely congruent with the idea of Minimalism in that words that are spoken are found to be of far greater value and extremely lacking in the idle chatter of the day that could be both distracting to study but also result in extraneous and frivolous thought that is not serving the purposes of the spiritual path. Outsiders may bock at the concept, but the art of silence is imperative to enlightenment for some. It helps them to really hone in on their ambitions as a student of philosophy or the tenets of their leaders. This too is important for cutting down on the instance of discussion where there could be unsavory or less-than-worthy topics discussed too, which is how it lends well to Minimalist thought.

Some believe that this practice has an imperative place in many spiritual trains of thought because it helps people to gain wisdom, center themselves, live in the present moment, enjoy life and contemplate things in a more poignant manner. This most certainly applies to Minimalism on all levels and can be found in some form in all religions as well as simple living. We all have times that we like to duck out and be silent within ourselves and retreat to some place where there is quiet around and within.

Enjoyment of the Simplicity in Life

One of the most interesting concepts I ever came across in all of my reading was also the most strange. When we start thinking about how Minimalism helps us to enjoy the smallest and simplest of joys in life, one particular item came to mind. Like a lot of people who delve deep into spiritual study, I read the book The Celestine Prophecy by James Redfield. In the book, the characters travel to an area in South America where there is a monastery. They encounter monks and enjoy a meal with them. While enjoying the meal, they notice that the monks are making a point to chew each bite of food 17 times before swallowing. Puzzled, the characters in the book question this practice, finding that the monks are savoring each flavor, texture and experience of the meal with every motion of their mouths.

This is but another example of the simple pleasures in life we absolutely take for granted in Western Civilization because we simply don't have the time or find it a laborious process to count or take extra time to think and feel. However, in this, you may yourself find a simplistic view of the world and your dining experience, learn to enjoy the company with you for your meal and even notice subtleties in your meal you could not before. Let's face it, a lot of people can't find time to make their own food these days let alone chew 17 times before swallowing. Our fast food generation is lucky to slide a meal down its gullets in more than 15 minutes before we're onto the next more-important task of the day.

There are examples of this even within weight loss counselling where it is advised to eat more slowly because in our society we eat so fast that we don't even notice when we're full. Just think on that for a second. We eat so fast that we don't even know when we've had enough –mindlessly shoveling it in until the plate or box is emptied because that more tells us we are done and can move on than our own bodies!

My question is: wouldn't it be lovely to embrace each meal and understand how wonderful it is that we can enjoy variety, tastes, spices, ingredients and all that goes into the making of what we put into our bodies? The Minimalist lifestyle challenges us to do just that and actually take these experiences and embrace them to the fullest because a meal really is a blessing, isn't it? The monks encountered in The Celestine Prophecy certainly demonstrated this aptly for me, and I know it will make sense for each of you if you do so the next time you sit down for your next meal with loved ones. It makes the most perfect sense.

Meditation: Enjoy the Silence

One of the more obvious yet elusive ways to enter into a Minimalist mindset for myself has been through meditative states. You can do this with guided meditations or go with quiet contemplation, be lead into a dream-like euphoria through music, use binaural beats or a plethora of different methods that you may or may not be familiar with. The world is vastly complicated, we are inundated with sound, over-stimulating visuals throughout our day, and a lot of us work in offices in front of screens all day long. It goes without saying a lot of the time that we need to have that peace of mind and time out at the end of our days to unwind and refocus our energies in a lower vibrational level.

One of the most relaxing experiences can be plugging in your headphones, turning on an app for meditation and listening to something as basic as a series of tones derived from Tibetan Singing Bowls or even just a Chakra Cleansing where the sounds literally move through your body and help you to realign your energies. Minimalists can often be found taking up these practices because they, again, encourage us to break the pattern of racing through each day prioritizing the things that clearly do not matter in favor of gentle and soul-nourishing experiences.

Meditation at home in a quiet corner is great if it's all you can accomplish, but take it a step further if you can and go out into nature every so often to listen to the birds sing and the wind rustle through the trees. I think sometimes we forget that we too are of this earth and need to come back to silence, enjoying Mother Nature's breath on our necks and how it feels to just be still.

If you find it difficult to delve into a state like this in the dead quiet of the day, binaural beats – brainwave technology through soundwaves transmitted via stereo headphones, can also put you in the correct state. For this, Theta waves are best as they put us in a higher spiritual state of mind. Others are more for sleep induction or for stress relief, which is still all well and good, but they won't be of much help if you're constantly dozing off.

There are meditations you can do for all kinds of purposes too, but regardless of your preferences, this is one undertaking Minimalists find to be immensely beneficial to their needs and aim. Loving Kindness,

Mindfulness, religious, chakra-cleansers, deep relaxation, sleep-inducers…Really, the list is endless. You can find so many through online searches, mobile apps, audio files and more. So go nuts with these to get in the correct mindset or just help push out the metal clutter. You'll feel much better after a hard day, and it can definitely help you to adopt the appropriate attitude for living a simpler more effective lifestyle akin to Minimalism.

Becoming a Self-Imposed Yoga Master

Minimalists also find joy in the simplicity of taking care of their bodies well. This is of utmost importance because they understand that one's health is paramount to maintaining a simple life free of health complications that can mean added stress. One way that this folds into the spiritual realm is through regular practice of yoga. Yoga has many different varieties, which can be important to choose wisely from. There are gentle forms of yoga used to simply de-stress that are easier on the body such as Hatha while others enjoy the fitness aspect of it by practicing flow yoga, which involves moving from one position to the other (often with excellent flexibility and strength training) without a break until the end of a session.

Bikram yoga, often known as hot yoga, is another very popular type where practitioners will practice a variety of positions designed to test the body's limits while in heated environments to help cleanse the body and detoxify through sweating. However, no matter the variety you choose to undertake, you will find that each focuses on the use of breathing techniques, focusing on body awareness and an immense mind-body connection that is essential to being at one within ourselves.

This is very rarely seen in things like mindlessly jogging away on the treadmill where positioning isn't always imperative or aimlessly lifting weights and thinking about whatever comes to mind. These are great fitness experiences in their own rite, but they do not offer the same grounded centeredness that yoga can offer.

In parts of South Asia, yoga is seen as a deeply holistic spiritual practice that is absolutely linked to religion and revered for its use for thousands of years in both a fitness and religious capacity. Minimalists can gain insight from this with the knowledge that they are clearing their minds, again, of the daily mental clutter of life while nourishing the spirit. Fitness is a great byproduct of this that can be also enjoyed, but it is the simplicity of working one's body without any more than a mat, one's body and surroundings. Outdoor practices are even more enticing because they provide the connection with nature, rush of air whipping around oneself and feeling the sun on one's face as they pay homage to their bodies in a most attentive and respected manner, calling to the Higher Self for wisdom, retreat and replenishment that cannot be found just anywhere.

The Vow of Poverty

As has been mentioned over and over again, Minimalist living is definitely not about how many possessions you own, but the fact of the matter is that there is an undertone of lack of possessions when we further examine how people choose to observe this lifestyle. Whether it be through décor schemes within the home, lack of owning a TV, living in smaller spaces or simply taking off and owning what can fit in a backpack or on the shelf of whichever hostel they choose to stay at, Minimalism does often take on the position of owning less or at least owning things of value as opposed to many things of frivolous proportions.

From a spiritual or religious aspect, this is most commonly seen with vows of poverty where those practicing Christianity that are deeper in their faith such as monks, priests and nuns would move into their parishes and abandon all possessions, wear only the clothing of their faith's requirement, devote their lives to service in the name of their creator and own nothing more than the Holy Bible, a rosary and their name –sometimes less than that. Despite what many believe, this isn't all that common anymore in Western Civilization with the new generation of definitions when it comes to devoting oneself to God, but it does still reach heights of prevalence in some pockets of our neck of the wood. In Eastern Civilization, many devout followers of other religions still observe vows of poverty and others are thrust into poverty without a choice in the matter to begin with.

Regardless, it's still a good to make a point of

shrugging off a lot of your 'things' in an effort to examine what is most important in your life to keep and what doesn't factor into your happiness at all. No one needs that much stuff anyway, but you may find that when you unshackle yourself of the chains of owning possessions, you also free yourself of unwanted and unnecessary debt, can enable yourself to live in a smaller home and even become a lot more unencumbered by societal norms associated with keeping up with the Joneses. Filling your life with experiences is by far more fulfilling than adding more items to it. I think most Minimalists will attest to this quite passionately.

If you're not big on doing so or have a hard time letting go of things you do own, you can start off small by eliminating unnecessary purchases first and then branch out by ridding your home of unwanted or outdated items you have no sentimental or personal attachments to. Go step by step in baby steps and you may find it easier than you once thought. If you're a bit more bold, you can move into a smaller place and sell off a bunch of stuff to start or have a garage sale every year to rid your home of all the clutter chaining you down and overcrowding your home.

Another perfect way to observe a modern-day vow of poverty of sorts is to stop being so trend-focused in matters of fashion. Start discount shopping or checking out thrift shops for your furniture and clothing to see what kinds of things you can grab at a fairly decent rate. Or limit your wardrobe to key pieces instead of doing the whole walk-in closet thing.

A lot of women love their shoes, but maybe you can go with a pair of runners, a pair or two of pumps, a pair of boots and some sandals. To be honest, a lot of my office colleagues already admittedly jump straight into pajamas the moment they get home from work, so it's not like we have a million outfit changes a day. Don't be a slave to the mindset that you have to keep all those clothes when there are plenty of people who can't clothe themselves as it is. Go through your closet every so often and donate all the things that don't fit or you aren't wearing to charity. Who cares what you purchased it for? If you aren't going to wear it, it's simply taking up space and another item bogging you down!

Okay, so we're totally going off on a tangent that only sort of relates to the actual vow of poverty taken on by religious folks, but it does absolutely make sense to adopt these behaviors if you're aim is a Minimalist lifestyle. Catholicism in particular takes this on in the fashion of owning nothing privately but for the common good of all and their religion only. This is to the extreme side of the spectrum, but it most certainly illustrates the point of simplicity and to which degree it simplifies life for those who observe it.

Chapter Three: Guilt by Association – You are Who You Hang With

Our mothers all warned us as children to be weary of the people we hung out with, didn't they? They always told us that we were who we hung out with, and although we may have initially ignored this fact, it is just that: fact. You can't associate with yuppies and not be a yuppie yourself. Just like you can't avoid the label of criminal when your best friends are thieves, druggies or hardcore criminals themselves.

This inconvenient fact makes it difficult to enjoy life when you have to cut fun people out of your like –while one can find it hard to imagine how shady people would be considered *fun* to chill with. But still, it's true, and the Minimalist lifestyle definitively calls for simplicity in your relationships with others in addition to the other things you might want to limit or stave off from altogether.

Ditching Stress-Inducing Relationships

While still an extremely challenging task, it is

imperative to ensure you are doing your best to rid yourself of stress-inducing relationships if you want to truly embrace Minimalism. It's nice to be there for people when they need you, but some individuals take advantage far too much, which isn't necessarily the most practical or relaxing.

It's not easy to take a step back and see your relationships for what they really are –just like looking at yourself long and hard in the mirror and seeing your own flaws. However, you must not be one of those individuals who constantly allows yourself to be pulled into codependent relationships where there is far too much drama and everything you care about takes a backseat to what others are going through.

I know many friends who have left their careers on the backburner, waiting for their spouses to finally get that job that was the perfect fit only to find that years later they were still waiting for their husband or wife to get their lives together –and they still had nothing to show for their lives. The same goes for abuse. Sticking around and waiting for people to change when they clearly are looping back around to the same behaviors they were guilty of in the first place is a waste of time. Who knows how long we have left on this planet, and decades can go by in a flash without one noticing just how much time has been wasted waiting for things to get better or someone to finally see the light.

On a very serious note, if you are suffering from abuse in your home or relationships, getting out is the only option. With that being said, the focus on minimizing your relationships has a broader meaning than just getting rid of the scumbags that tend to latch onto good people who are willing to give of themselves so freely. Minimalists will pick and choose quality people to have in their lives that are supportive, non-judgmental and worthy of forming tight bonds with. After all, we may have just the one ride on the Merry-Go-Round, so it is of utmost importance to realize that decluttering your lives of sour, unhealthy and superficial relationships is key to leading a Minimalist track of mind.

You don't need to be immediately visceral about it, but it really helps to make sure that you're at least weaning yourself off codependent relationships that thrive on the *Drama Triangle* paradigm that shifts onus from one person to the other for every issue life throws at them. If you're unfamiliar with this concept, it works like so: one person is the aggressor, another the victim and the remaining, the rescuer.

When you or someone you know has issues with codependency, you will recognize the drama triangle is a regular part of their make-up. They cannot accept responsibility for their part in the problem, won't acknowledge where they can make changes to improve the situation, and can't keep out of other conflicts because there is an innate need to insert themselves into the fray to fall into, at the very least, the rescuer role.

A lot of families and romantic relationships have codependency within them, which is a shame because those trying to move into a Minimalist mindset can often be pulled right back into this triangle –even against their wishes. The point is to understand how this is happening and to distance yourself from these sorts of relationships so you can understand that the focus should be on those who do not expect nor thrust you into a category or role that is both emotionally and mentally draining.

Unfortunately, this may mean disowning parents who have addiction issues, spouses who are abusive or aren't pulling their weight but limiting your ability to be happy and so many more energy vampires that just want to take your energy and power away from you. The same goes for friends! We all have a few friends who only come around when they need something or when things in their lives seem to be going awry.

Support is one thing, but you have to maintain a healthy balance in their lives of peace, calm and sensitivity. You can't hang around people who only complain or go into sympathetic overdrive about the minute issues that are bothering them all the time. If so, there wouldn't be much time left in your days to devote to those who matter most like your children, lover, work relationships and more.

Minimalism specifically calls for you to rid your life of people and things that no longer serve you in a positive manner. This is absolutely an important step in simplifying your living. There have to be boundaries as to what and whom you will tolerate in this arena, so don't be afraid to slowly stop calling or hanging out with those who suck you dry of your time and energy with little benefit to your ideals and path in life. Again, you are who you associate with, so keep this in mind when you go out and how each person you allow in your life makes you feel. If this doesn't seem to fit well, don't force it but move away from it in an effort to keep your peace of mind intact.

Social Networking and its Impact on Minimalism

To be perfectly honest with you, Social Media is a fantastic networking tool and Rolodex of sorts for finding people you want to reach out to. It doesn't have to mean you are constantly inundating yourself with relationships with people who don't have any relevance to your life or those you've drifted apart from. What is does mean is that you should not allow people on your Friends Lists that you do not know or have only met online. Keep it to people you want to or could see yourself wanting to reach out to moving forward. Don't feel bad for doing some housecleaning and removing acquaintances you barely know (or that catfish that's been messing with you or stalking your profile incessantly).

While this may be completely up to you and absolutely permissible, you don't need to be a massive dick about it. There is no need to twist the knife in and publicly ensure certain people are 'not important' enough to be a part of your lists. Maintain equilibrium and remember that several people in your list of over 300 friends may not have a necessity to view your posts or aren't cool enough for you. What it really means is that you can remove people, but be mindful of the impending repercussions of removing a person or two when it could result in upsetting feelings of rejection and be quite hurtful on a bad day.

A lot of Minimalists will ditch their Social Media accounts in an effort to limit the amount of daily appeasement via Likes, Shares or reposts. In fact, it's more than just the Minimalist that does so. A lot of people have had to ditch Social Media because it is a massive distraction to their personal relationships in real life, takes up far too much time to maintain and can be an all-consuming portion of life although it lives completely in the intangible. So I invite all those attempting to observe the Minimalist lifestyle to rid themselves of the responsibility of

Social Media to remove the complications associated with it. Unplugging, you will find, can be an extremely liberating feeling.

Invite Positivity Into Your Circle Instead

With all of this talk about elimination of things and people, there are still a lot of things you should invite into your life when observing a Minimalist lifestyle. One of the biggest things you will want to do when addressing your personal relationships is making a point to recognize and embrace those personal relationships you have with individuals who have immense positive energy or are supportive in your ambitions, challenges and life in general. Having a circle of friends (big or small, but typically smaller) has a positive impact on your life and can activate change in you to become a more positive and happy person yourself.

The simplicity in this comes effortlessly when you find the right people to be around. They do not expect anything from you –you can come away from your interactions with them full well knowing that there are no heavy-duty expectations placed on you.

That you owe them nothing. Unconditional love in romantic relationships, supportive friendships, family dynamics that allow you to be who you are unencumbered –these are all great examples of the kinds of relationships that Minimalists enjoy once they've rid themselves of the negative influences in their lives.

Even relationships with coworkers who celebrate your successes with you and fully admonish you to follow your ambitions are a huge motivator. These are the kinds of people you may need to hunt for for a long time; they are few and far between, but they can absolutely revolutionize your outlook and help you along the way like sentinels, validating your good decisions and uplifting you to empowerment. Seek these people out and make sure you have your tribe with you and you will be set for life. Minimalism calls for these things to be more of a focus than the money you earn and the possessions you keep because they are so much more valuable and fulfilling –replenishing to your soul.

The Ripple Effect of Negativity and Your Role Within It

While reading the book *Stepping Up* by John Izzo, a wonderful point was immediately brought up when discussing the Pillars of Responsibility. While Minimalism itself focuses on uncomplicating life so that you can live freely and enjoy life to the fullest for every drop, there is great responsibility that must be taken in your relationships for your part within them. You can and should surround yourself with those who are supportive, sensitive to your needs, positive and harmonious within your circle, but you must also accept responsibility for your role within these as well.

It was very apparent when reading on that the most important thing one can do is step up and ensure that their part in each interaction is something each individual holds themselves accountable to. I am only happy because I so choose to be, and if you are in a group of people and someone complains or rants on and on about a bad day or negative experience, this has a ripple effect that causes others to do the same or take on the negativity themselves.

This is not unlike tossing a pebble into a pond

and watching the ripples in the water move further out and on until dispersing into the rest of the pond. So when you interact with your peers, friends and family, ensure that you are taking responsibility for your part in these and how you can create your own ripple effect too.

Minimalists tend to be more peaceful human beings because of the simplistic lifestyle they've began to observe, but this doesn't mean we all don't have bad days. When and if you do, be aware of the urge to blurt it all out to the world and how that will impact those around you. If you're doing it right, you can exude and demonstrate some extremely bright and lighthearted energy that can be just as contagious as the negative garbage a lot of other people may throw out into the universe. Simplify your feelings and how you communicate them as well, and you find that you can better articulate how you feel and how you wish to enact change and happiness in your personal relationships in the world at large.

You Can't Run from Your Family, or Can You?

Family is a huge part of everyone's life. You can run away, you can disown them, you can tell them you need to live your own life, but they will always be there. Truth is, your family is engrained in you. In psychology, they call it conditioning. Others describe it as being a product of their environments. To the contrary of the Minimalist, my father is a massive pack rate, and my sister spoils her step children with oodles of gifts to make up for the time they were away. I don't live in the same area of the nation as my family, but they are a part of who I am.

Yes, you can't run from your family. However, you can revolutionize those relationships to simplify them and make sure that they are understanding your change to a better, more positive and immensely simplified life. Your immediate family may not understand. Mom will definitely need a total breakdown of the concept and reminders on what it all actually means, but if they're able to, they will most certainly support your efforts to move into a Minimalist ideal.

If you are the patriarch or matriarch of your own

by now, you can instill the Minimalist Lifestyle in your own family as well. Start right away with your children so they know no different. It doesn't have to be extreme as we all well know that kids are very trend-focused and need to stay up-to-date on all the things all their friends have, but you can still do simple diets, minimal toys or possessions, less TV time, avoiding social media as long as possible, sharing of experiences instead of money and so much more.

Kids never remember that time that mom and dad bought XYZ, but they absolutely remember and cherish the time you spend and the effort you put in to ensure they are in your company. In other cultures, parents have far better attachments with their children, which only goes to benefit the child-parent relationship. It can be as simple as a daily walk together or gathering around the TV for a Sunday afternoon movie. Minimalist lifestyles call for less clutter and fewer things and more time for the things that matter, and your kids need to know that they matter. Your work will still be there in an hour, but children are only children for so long and then they're gone off into the world. This is something to embrace without a doubt!

Chapter Four: You are What You Eat too!

The simplicity of Minimalism can be far-reaching, and it touches regions of your life such as food too. With all the processed crap lining the shelves of grocery stores these days, it's pretty standard for a Minimalist to want to eliminate all of the junk out of their diet and stick to clean eating; especially when the benefits are so clear. Sure, at first it won't seem so great. You're going to miss a lot of the added salt, sugar, artificial flavorings and other garbage they pack into a lot of the snacks you're used to enjoying.

After a while, your taste buds will adapt and you'll begin to really enjoy –even celebrate the foods you're eating without them. Clean eating is a huge part of a Minimalist lifestyle because it helps you to save money in some capacities but also shows you how to respect your body, prolonging your life and helping you to live a happier and more fulfilling existence since you won't be full of chemicals and other additives through food.

No, You Don't Have to Be a Vegan…

By now, you're likely to be used to the idea that there are a lot of common misconceptions about Minimalism. Yes, these blend into eating as well. One of the most prevalent of these is the idea that all Minimalists are Vegans. No. They are not all Vegans. In fact, all you have to do is eat clean! Of course, there are a lot of Minimalists who do believe that following a Vegan diet is best for them, but that's a separate ideal far from the Minimalist Lifestyle with its own beliefs that have to do with animal cruelty, personal preferences, diet restrictions and so much more that doesn't typically involve Minimalism itself.

If you do choose to follow a Vegan lifestyle to rid yourself of the meat portion of your diet, that's purely up to you. However, be aware that there are a few things that make this a bit more complicated than one would initially think. There are a lot of differentiations between levels of Veganism. There are people who simply do not eat meat. There are others who do not eat meat but also avoid eggs and dairy as well. Then there are others who take it as far as not wearing or consuming anything that has to do with animal products at all. This means no leather, nothing that was tested on animals and literally everything that ever had to do with an animal being involved in its production whatsoever.

As you can see, that can get super complicated if you start looking at all the research and detours in the supermarket, with cosmetics, furniture, clothing and so much more. I mean, if you have those convictions, definitely stick by them; good on you for being so committed to your cause, but if you want to live a Minimalist lifestyle and aren't already doing the Vegan thing, this may be a fairly arduous process for you that you don't really want to delve into. It doesn't mean it isn't a worthy cause, but it does require a lot of work, which stricter Vegans can absolutely attest to when addressing those who are just starting out and have no clue about what it's all about.

Simple Eating and its Health Benefits

Eating a simpler and cleaner diet of fresh foods that aren't processed through factories and stuffed with additives and preservatives has a ton of helath benefits that most Minimalists will readily attest to.

You'll feel less bogged down, have far more energy, notice your digestion runs a lot smoother, have better sleep patterns if you quell your caffeine intake, notice some weight loss if that's been an issue and generally feel far better. Your skin will even start to look better with fewer breakouts, a healthier glow and more.

Just stick to a diet rich in fruits, vegetables, protein in the form of meats, nuts and seeds, whole grains instead of the refined variety of carbs and you'll definitely notice that shopping trips are easier and your body feels tons better than it used to. As a former weight loss counsellor, I can tell you right now that it is always recommended to ditch prepackaged garbage in favor of the simpler fare. If you didn't want to get up and move before, you will after your body gets used to enjoying all those meal options instead of processed trash.

That is exactly what it is too, processed crud that goes through a ton of different chemical treatments to rid it of a bunch of stuff, then they have the audacity to run it through even more processing to re-add back all of the nutrients boiled and processed out of it just so it's considered 'good for you' again. Let me tell you right now, any nutrient added back to your food is more than likely synthetic or processed out of something else in a lab. What would be better than putting food into your body that has the nutrients in it to begin with rather than having it go through the wringer just to have everything added back in?

This should be common sense, but because most people are far too busy to notice or care, we just pick up whatever we can find that has healthy buzzwords on its packaging and believe it to be the best option, and deep down, we know that isn't the truth. Because Minimalists have simpler lives and the time to devote to things that matter, they can take the time to make a trip to the local farmer's market, butcher shop or spend additional time in the produce portion of their supermarket to get quality foods that help with health issues or prevent them. Eating healthier diets in general has proven time and again to prevent all manner of health issues from the common cold all the way to cancer. You can't argue with that!

The 100-Mile Diet…Is it That Simple?

A lot of people who reexamine their diets have come across the concept of the 100-Mile Diet. This is a great concept for a lot of people –and it does make sense for a lot of people who really want to curb their use of foods that are massively processed and contain a lot of preservatives and other disgusting additives, but is it that simple of an undertaking? That's the real question you have to ask yourself if you're looking at the Minimalist lifestyle and your diet.

The 100-Mile Diet is very easy to follow in theory. You really only have to follow one rule: only consume foods that are produced within 100 miles of your residence. That's a very noble idea! Living in a coastal region, this can afford people the ability to enjoy seafood, fresh produce and more, but it doesn't cover all the bases. You're never going to eat chocolate again unless you live in Africa or South America –just to be clear. Salt is going to be something you have to make via the distillation process (if you live near the ocean), and you'll need to relearn how to create leavening unless you live near a baking powder/soda factory.

In fact, you might find yourself traveling to the outer edges of that 100 miles to get some of the things necessary for a healthy diet, and unless you plan on being perfect, you're going to slip and have a cup of coffee from time to time. Of course, you can be hard on yourself and follow the tenets of the diet to the letter, but it's really not that simple if you're in an area that grows corn and raises livestock but couldn't produce a peach if hell froze over.

Another issue is that in the modern world, we have the luxury of having produce year-round due to the convenience of shipping produce from other more tropical locales that can provide this during the Winter to us when we have nothing green living outside. It will encourage you to garden and can more of your produce, but what are you to do if you have children? How are you to sustain a proper nutritional balance for yourself if you aren't able acquire specific foods in your area? If you're an apathetic person not willing to do the research or other legwork, you're definitely in for a shock with this 100-Mile Diet concept.

So before you throw out everything in your cupboards and declare yourself a proponent to this idea, make sure you look around, have a search of what you can and cannot get in your area, and ensure you're able to really commit to what it means. It won't be a walk in the park (unless you're foraging), so ask yourself: would a Minimalist embrace this? If the answer for you is yes, then do a ton of research and don't be lazy in your goal to stick with it. Otherwise, you're just setting yourself up for failure, which you most likely don't want to go through.

If you're worried about processed foods, just stick to the outer rim of the grocery store and get your meals from there instead. I apologize if this sounds defeatist, but I'm a realist, and I know that it's not practical nor feasible in a lot of living situations, geographical areas or for some people's lifestyles. SO why complicate matters with more when you're essentially trying to simplify everything for yourself. It's just counterintuitive to the whole thing and very counterproductive as well.

Drugs, Toxins and How They Affect Your Path

Yeah, I know that drugs aren't necessarily foods, but you have to take note: Minimalists don't generally put anything in their bodies that's going to complicate their lives. Clean eating is one thing, but this also extends into other things we put into our bodies. Everything in moderations, right? So don't go heavy on the alcohol. It will only damage your liver and make for bad choices, which as adults, we should all be well aware of anyway, but even so. Don't drink too much!

Aside from drinking, there are those who feel that there are drugs you can take in your travels to reach *enlightenment*. SO not true! Taking drugs is dangerous. It's not good for your body, relationships, career or lifestyle in general; it works to the contrary of a Minimalist lifestyle, wreaking havoc on your judgment, body and complicates your life with all sorts of mistakes you may not have otherwise made, costs a lot of money and could even result in addiction. Not to mention it is a serious health risk these days with the advent of Fentanyl-laced substances, overdoses, psychological effects and more. So do as the PSAs say and avoid this garbage at all costs. Mic drop!

Chapter Five: In Summation

So with all of this info that you're now armed with, you have a general understanding of what Minimalism is and is not, correct? It's not just about junking your TV, ditching your car or deciding to go on that pilgrimage across Europe. You can still do all those things. Sure, go nuts! But the paramount idea here is to simply live simply. Do so unencumbered; lose the relationships in your life that are creating massive issues for you. Stop inviting circumstances and items into your space that make you feel stressed out or clutter up your life with too many things or problems.

Of course, life is never without its hiccups as it is, but you can lessen those by following all these key principles, allowing yourself to drop the major weights in your life in favor of living for what is most important and truly focusing in on those things. Because let's face it, life really is too short, isn't it? Your job will be there when you get up tomorrow morning, so spend more time with your loved ones. Turn your phones to mute every so often and really take in nature when you go out into your city's green space. Heck, move out of the city and onto an acreage or opt for a more peaceful existence through practices such as meditation.

Release yourself from the pressures of keeping up with modern trends because you don't need a TV that's 50 inches when you already own a 42 inch. Why buy that tablet when you have a laptop and phone? How many pairs of shoes do you honestly need? Start examining your own life for where you could eradicate debt, problematic piles of junk you never look at that take up space in closets and corners of your home, overstimulating living spaces, relationships that are pointless and going nowhere… there are so many things we allow ourselves to go through, participate in or own that we really don't need.

Far more important things, places and experiences await us all in life; the knowledge of this alone is enough to begin your own Minimalist path now. As little or as extreme as you want to take it, you will find yourself feeling more lighthearted, relaxed and upbeat. If you have a smaller home, you won't need that second job, and if you opt to ease off socializing with those 150 friends on social media, you might have more time for your children and the other people in your life that matter more than fair-weather friends or acquaintances that don't do anything but demand more of your time when they bring nothing to the table.

The responsibility and choice is yours, but with all that has been shared and all that you can experience that awaits you around each and every corner in your life as you eliminate more and more of the 'stuff' you don't need, you will most certainly come to truly live in greater appreciation for what the world has to offer you –and that's a lot. It's freedom, it's happiness and its true beauty –a quality of life you may have never imagined. It's never been so easy as this. It's virtually effortless.

Live in that knowing and you will learn the true joy of Minimalism.